Vince Gironda's

A Muscle Has

FOUR SIDES

How To Build More Muscle In the Shortest Time Possible.

(Print Replica. Lite Editing for Acuity, and Clarity)

AL Rock with VinceGirondaNaturalBodybuilding.Com

VINCE GIRONDA'S

A Muscle Has FOUR SIDES

(Print Replica)

Be sure to leave an honest review after you read this book! I would appreciate it greatly.

Vincent Anselmo Gironda (November 9, 1917 – October 18, 1999)

HALL OF FAME – VENICE MUSCLE BEACH – 2016

Check out this book's official Website and YouTube Chanel

VinceGirondaNaturalBodyBuilding.Com

AL Rock with VinceGirondaNaturalBodybuilding.Com

A MUSCLE HAS FOUR SIDES

How To Build More Muscle In The Shortest Time Possible.

Vince Gironda

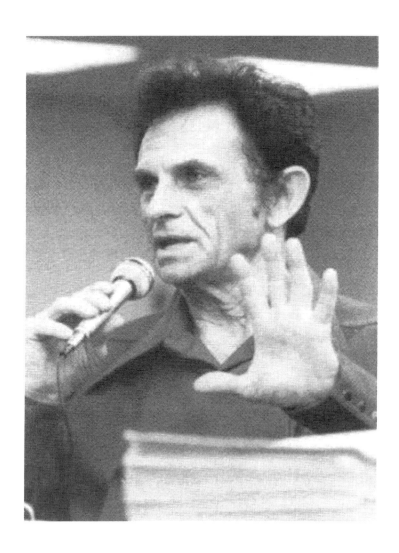

"When Vince Speaks the Stars Listen"

A MUSCLE HAS FOUR SIDES

How To Build The Most Muscle Size In The Shortest Time Possible

Introduction

All the concepts I have advanced over the years have initially met with a certain amount of skepticism, usually because initially they seem too simple to achieve the results desired in the time given. Yet eventually, sometimes twenty-five years later, these concepts are accepted around the world as standard training axioms. I will tell you now what the secret of success really is. Believe that the course I give will work, and it will. If you have doubts, and don't put everything into it, then you will find it won't work. The following course, A Muscle Has Four Sides, is based upon the fact that different exercises develop different parts of a given muscle. By doing four exercises, one for each part of the muscle, you will achieve the fastest possible growth. Combine this with proper workout frequency, and correct nutrition that I give you, and the muscle will grow at the fastest possible rate. Doing more will not improve results, in fact if you do the exercises properly, you will not be able to do more. I am currently training a Mr. Universe winner with 20 years experience, and he tells me that this is the most difficult routine he has ever done. Now on to the exact performance. Read every word several times before you start.

Exercise Style and Performance

Each exercise in this course is performed one set only and for 12 repetitions, with exception of the calves which are 20 repetitions. These are four different exercises for each muscle group. Before starting on a muscle group you set up the equipment required for all four exercises, so that you can move directly from one exercise to the next without delay. On each exercise you perform inter-muscular contractions, that is, tense the muscle voluntarily at the top of each movement. The principle here is the greatest amount of work done in the shortest period of time gets the greatest results. This is the reason sprinters have more leg muscle development than long distance runners, who do a lot more work. This concept pumps up the capillaries for increased muscle size. Additional exercises and sets would only cause overtonis, shock to the central nervous system, and loss of muscle size. As far as poundages go, you must force yourself to complete the required number of repetitions, even if this requires some cheating on the last two or three. However do not baby yourself by cheating too early in the set. Since all four exercises are performed consecutively, you naturally will be stronger on the first ones. It will probably take you a couple of workouts to adjust the poundages.

Exercise Frequency

This is a variation of the split routine, however you will workout twice each day, performing the same exercises in the second workout as you did in the first. The workouts must be separated by at least four hours, and in the second workout you may have to use slightly less poundages than the first. However, if you do be sure to use stricter style and tighter muscular contractions. These are the body parts you will work day by day in the following order:

- **Day 1- Back, Chest and Shoulders.**
- **Day 2- Triceps, Biceps and Forearms.**
- **Day 3- Thighs and Calves.**
- **Day 4- Same as Day 1.**
- **Day 5- Same as Day 2.**
- **Day 6- Same as Day 3**
- **Day 7- Rest.**

There is no abdominal work on this course. This is a muscle size building course and AB (abdominal) work can shock the solar plexus and slow down gains.

I have found that abdominals can be developed in six weeks, and if you wish to do this, order the complete course I have written.

The Routine, Day 1 – Back

Exercise 1 – Low Pulley Pull.

This exercise works two different parts of the Lats, the Teres Major, and the section of the Traps between the shoulder blades. Use a low pulley machine with the pulley 16" off the floor, and try about 120 to 150 pounds. Pull the bar from a full stretch position head down, until it touches just under the low pec line. Keep your elbows out wide, and at the completion of the movement your chest should be high, and the shoulders drawn down and back.

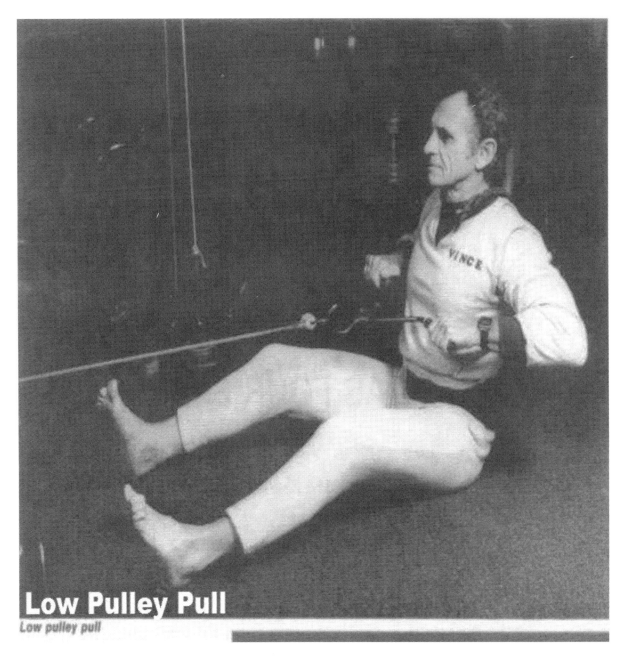

Low Pulley Pull

Low pulley pull

Exercise 2 – Reeves Alternate Rowing.

This exercise develops the Teres Muscles for width across the upper back at the shoulders. Lay two dumbbells on the floor with the handles parallel to each other. As the name implies, you perform alternate bent over rowing movements, pulling one dumbbell up with the elbow pointed straight out to the side as you lower the dumbbell. You must use intermuscular contraction, that is, keep all the muscles used tensed throughout the exercise.

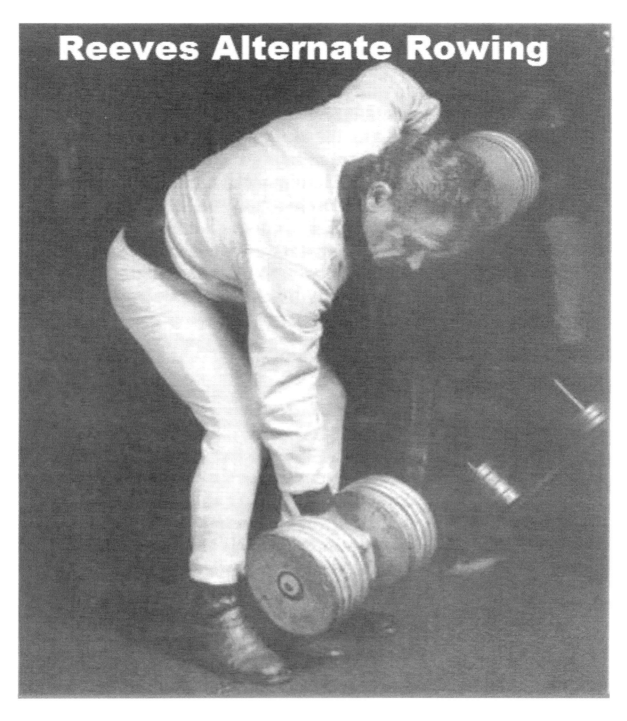

Exercise 3 – Low Pulley Rowing from Racing Dive Position.

This exercise will give you that Long Lat Sweep. Use the same pulley machine with the pulley 16" off the floor that you used in exercise 1. From a standing position, bend over and crouch in a racing dive position. The thighs and abdomen must be kept touching throughout the entire movement. Grasp the bar 16" wide and drop your head down between your arms. Pull the bar back to just under the low pec line, at the same time squeezing your shoulders back and down to contract the Lats. Keep your elbows out wide throughout the movement.

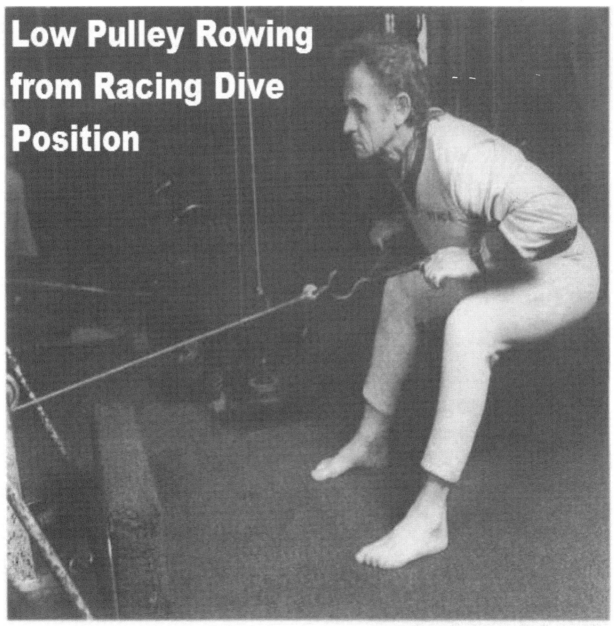

Low pulley rowing from racing dive position

Exercise 4 – Two Dumbbell Rowing.

Lying face down on a bench 20" high.

This exercise will thicken your upper back and bring out all the muscular detail. Place two heavy dumbbells on the floor under a flat bench 20" high, with the handles parallel. Lie on your stomach on the bench, and pull both dumbbells up as high as you can keeping your elbows out wide to the sides. As you pull the dumbbells up, lift your head and legs up, and arch your back. Between each repetition, lay the dumbbells on the floor and relax your grip. Use all the weight possible and still get a complete movement.

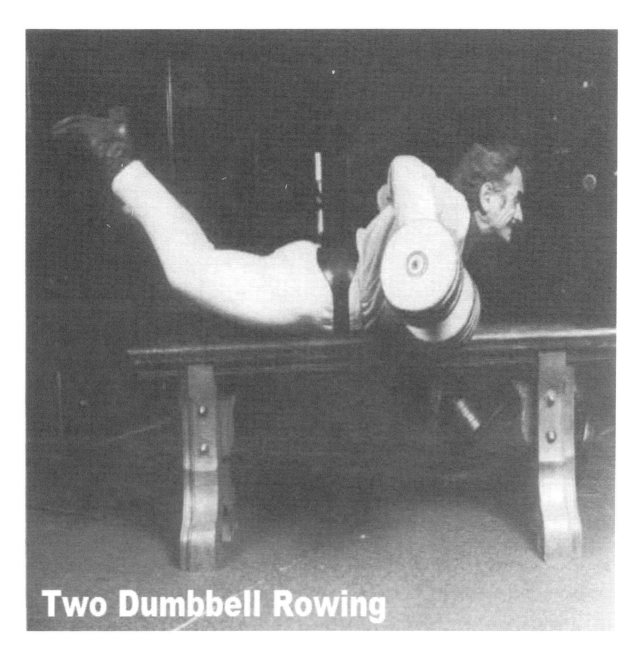

Two Dumbbell Rowing

Chest

Exercise 1 – Barbell Press to the Neck.

This exercise develops the Pectoralis Minor. Perform bench presses to the base of the neck with a medium wide hand spacing. Keep knees together and lower legs crossed throughout to isolate the movement.

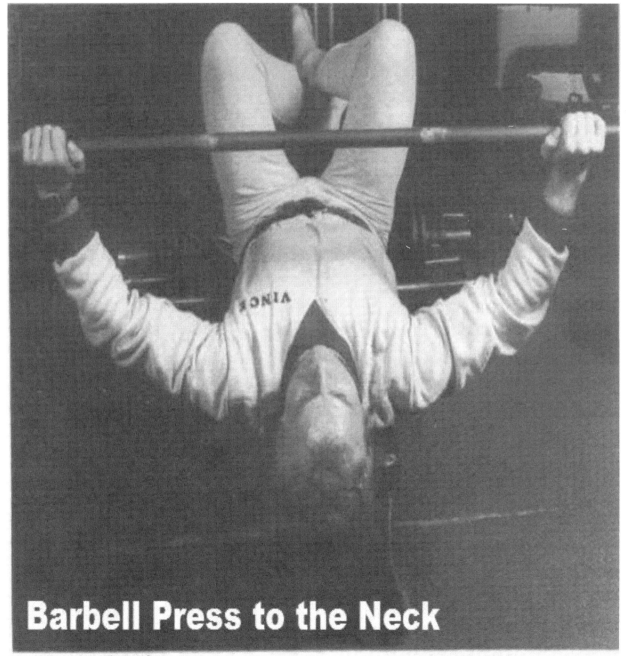

Barbell press to the neck

Exercise 2 – V Bar Dips.

This exercise will give you that lower and outer pec outline. Use a 32" wide grip, facing the V of the bar. Keep your chin on your chest, shoulders rounded forward, and elbows out wide to the sides throughout the movement. Point your toes down, keep them vertically below your face, and dip down as low as possible, then press up, maintaining your position. This is a difficult manner to dip, and if you can't make 12 full reps, push up the bottom 10 or 12 inches only until 12 counts are completed.

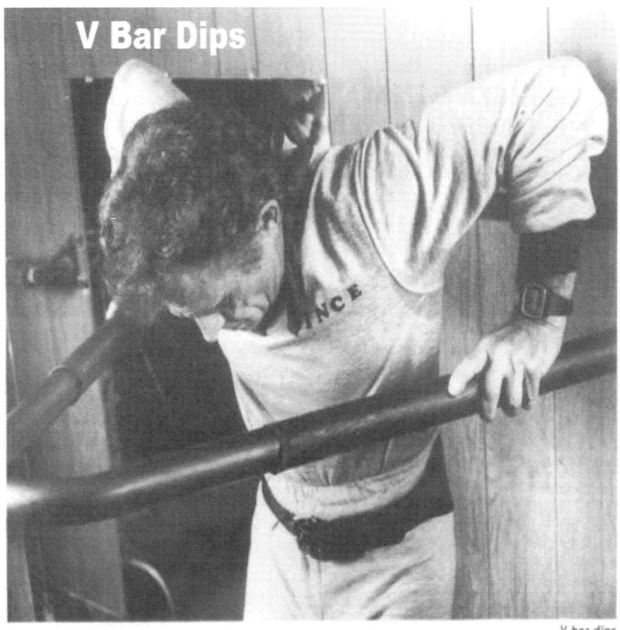

V bar dips

Exercise 3 – Incline Dumbbell Press.

For the Pectoralis Minor. Lying on the incline bench, press two dumbbells up until all four dumbbells touch together at the completion of the movement. The elbows must be kept out to the sides and the palms facing each other.

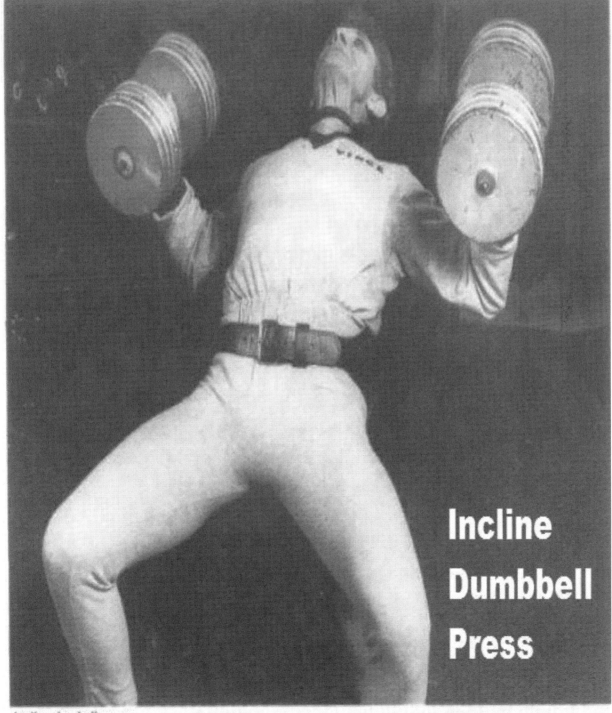

Incline dumbell press

Exercise 4 – Modified Bench Laterals.

This exercise is for the Middle Pectoral. Perform laterals with the palms facing each other while lying on a flat bench. Use a weight heavy enough that you have to bend your elbows, and perform a movement half-way between a full lateral and a press.

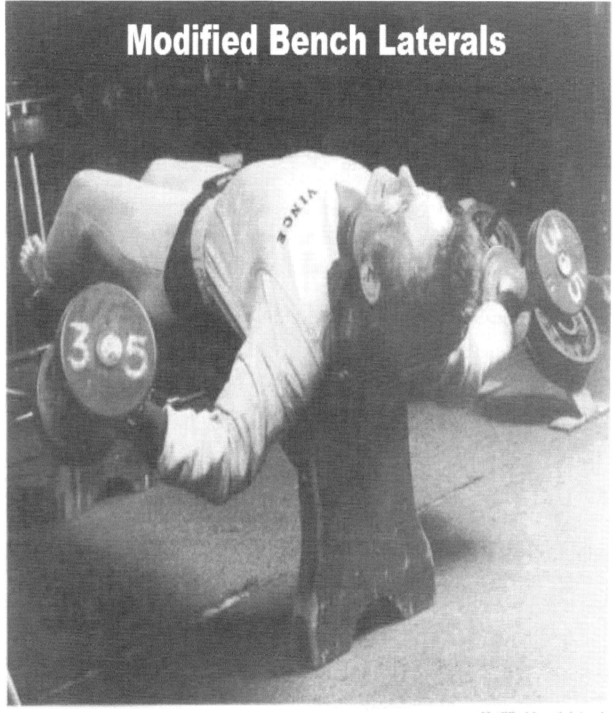

Modified bench laterals

Shoulders

Exercise 1 – Dumbbell DB Lateral Side Swing.

For the outside Part of the Deltoid. One arm is held out to the side slightly in front of the body (as in side lateral raise) and the other arm is held across and in front of the body, forearm in front of the face, palm down. Hold this contracted position for a second, then swing the dumbbells down in front of the body, and reverse the position of the arms. Do not twist the body.

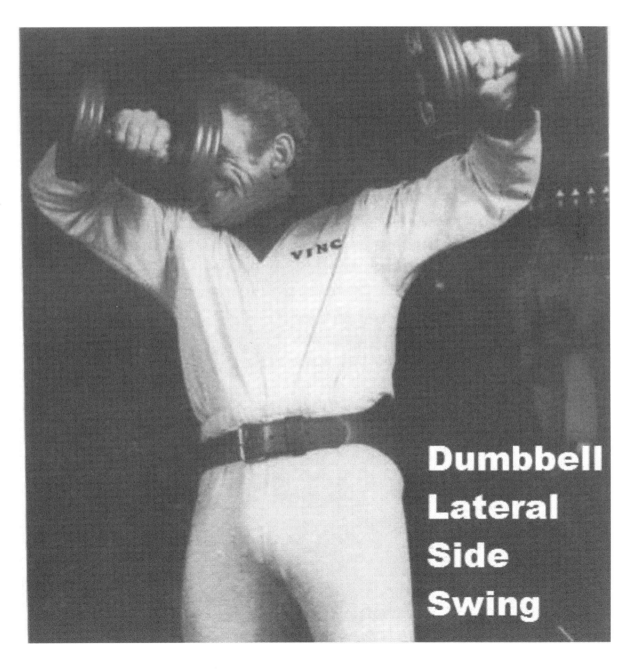

Dumbbell Lateral Side Swing

Exercise 2 – Barbell Upright Row.

This exercise develops the Lateral Deltoid where the Lateral and Posterior Heads meet. Use a shoulder width grip, and rest the barbell across the upper thighs. Lift the barbell, keeping the elbows high, to a position even with the upper chest, and about 12" in front. Hold in contracted position for a second before lowering.

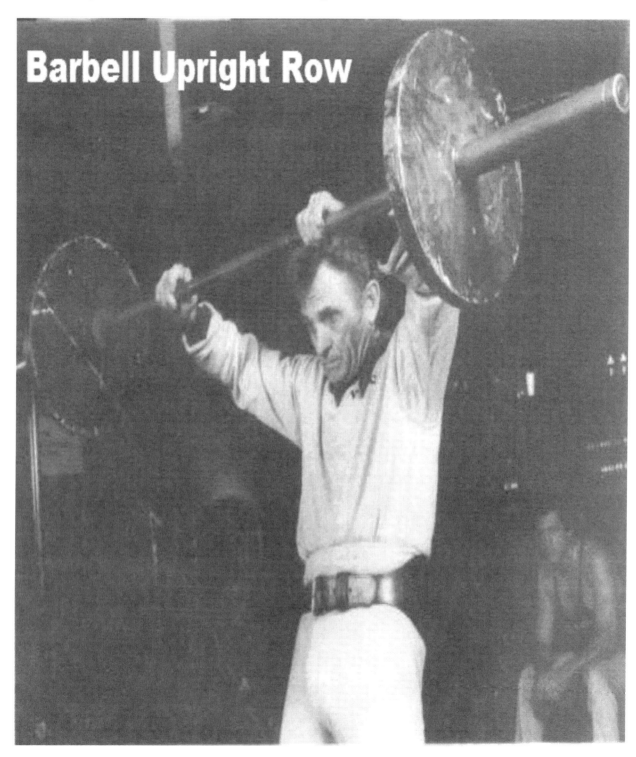

Exercise 3 – Scott Press.

For the Deltoid where the Anterior Head meets the Side. Hold two dumbbells together in front of the chest, with all four bells touching. Move the elbows out to the sides so that the dumbbells are in a wider than shoulder width position. Next, push the head forward and press the dumbbells up until they are even with the top of the head. Keep the palms forward. Reverse the movement and return to the starting position.

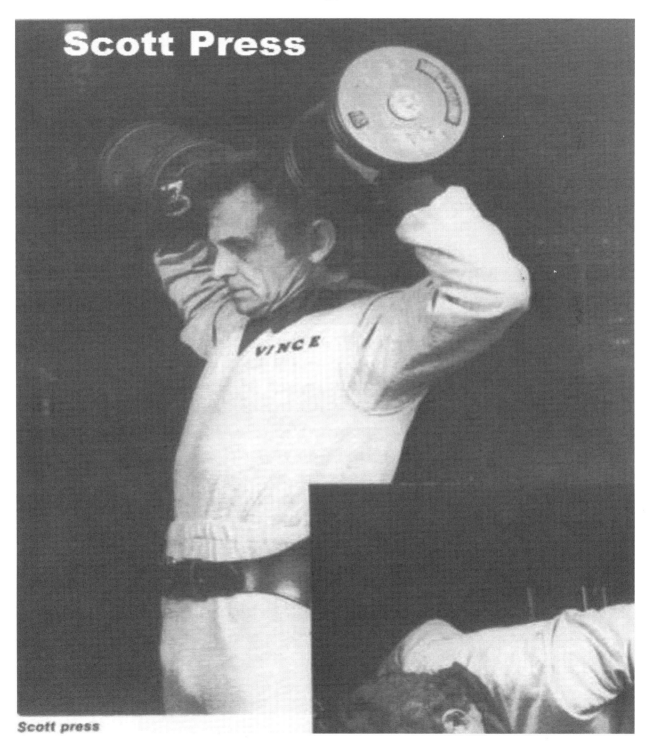

Scott press

Exercise 4 – Bent Over Dumbbell Laterals.

For the Rear Deltoid where it meets the Lateral Head. Stand bent over with a dumbbell in each hand, all four bells touching. Keep the head up and back arched. Lift the dumbbells directly out to the side, and at the top of the movement turn the front of the dumbbells slightly up. Pause in the contracted position, and lower slowly to the starting position. This completes your routine for Day 1.

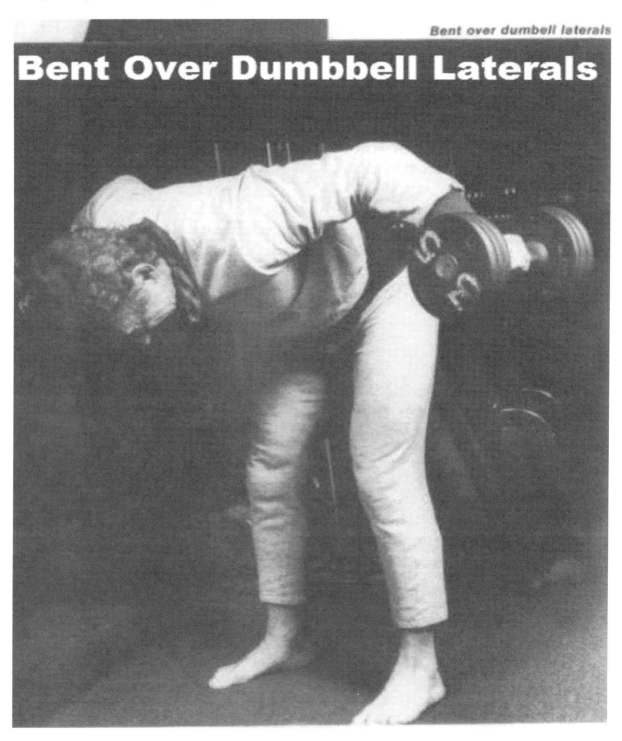

Day 2 – Triceps

Exercise 1 – Triceps Barbell Pull Over.

This exercise is for the Inner Tricep Head, between the elbow and shoulder. Lie on an exercise bench, with the top of your head over the bench and a barbell held at arms length over your chest. Your grip should be 12" wide. Keep your elbows in and lower the bar behind and just below your head. Return to starting position.

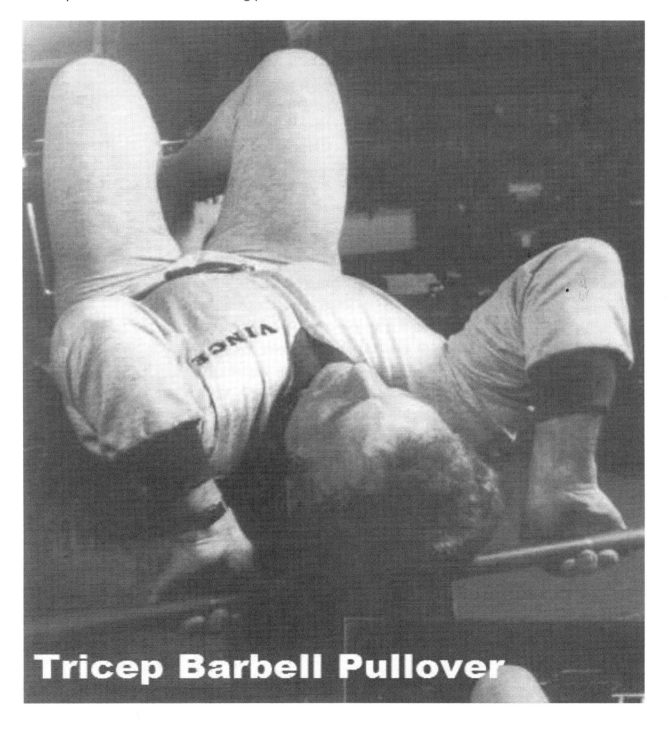

Tricep Barbell Pullover

Exercise 2 – Barbell Rollover and Press.

The pullover part of this exercise affects the High Tricep and the press the Outer Head. Lie on the same bench with the same body and head position as the previous exercise that is near the back of your head. From this position, pull the bar over close to your face, and rest it on your chest. Now rotate your elbows out to the sides, and press the bar to arms length over your chest. Try to press downward toward your feet to get a better contraction. Lower the bar to your starting position.

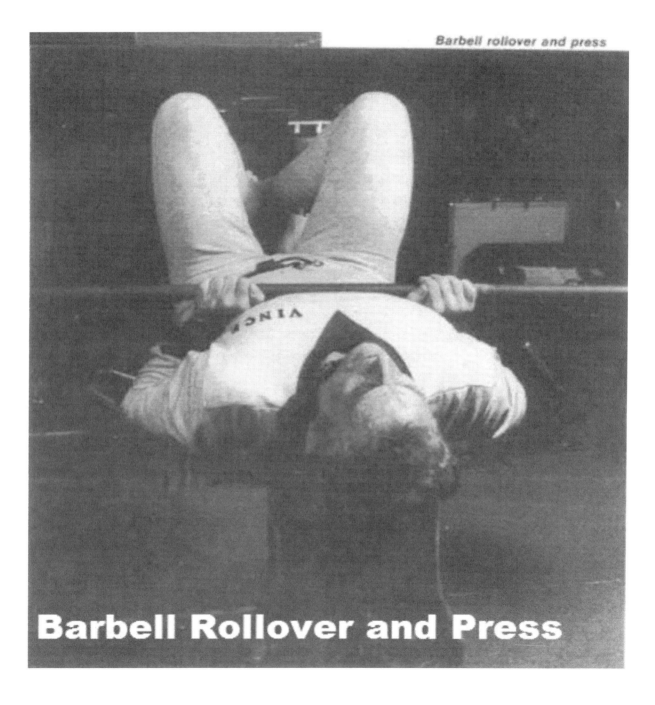

Barbell rollover and press

Barbell Rollover and Press

Exercise 3 – Reverse Close Parallel Dip.

For the High Head of the Triceps. This is not the same parallel dip given for chest in your Day 1 program. In this variation you face away from the V, if your parallel bars have a V, and dip with your chest out, back arched, head and feet back, and your elbows pointed to the rear. Be sure to lock out at the top of the movement.

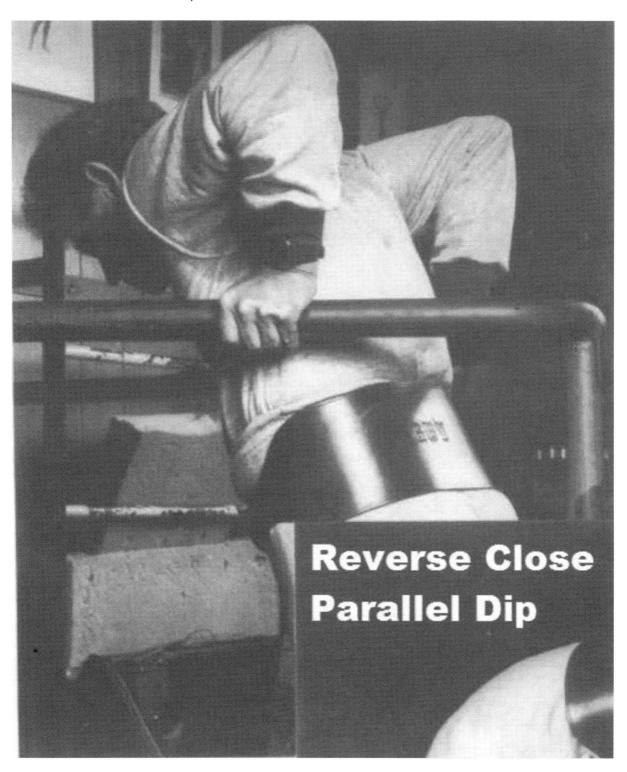

Reverse Close Parallel Dip

Exercise 4 – Dumbbell Kickback.

This exercise is for the High Head of the Tricep. Hold two dumbbells with the front ends touching your front delts. Bend over until your stomach and thighs are touching, your knees are bent. From this position, keeping your elbows still, straighten your arms. As you do so raise your hips slightly and lower your shoulders. Try to hold the contracted position for a second. Keep the elbows up, and return to the starting position.

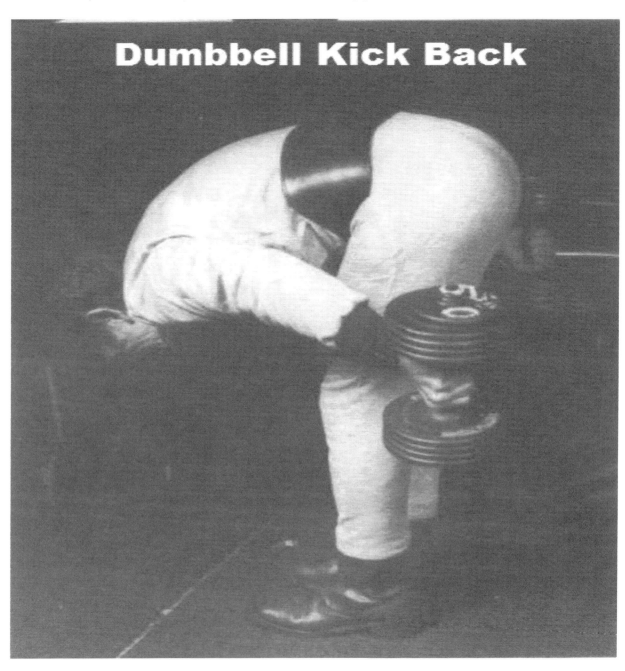

Biceps

Exercise 1 – Barbell Preacher Curl.

This exercise is for Low Biceps. Perform your preacher curls with the left foot forward under the bench, and the right foot back. Keep your stomach pressed against the elbow rest, and your head and shoulders inclined forward. Your grip should be shoulder width, and "thumb under". Close your fingers to a firm grip, bend your wrist up, and curl to the shoulders. Use smooth pumping reps, and do not lean back at the top of the movement.

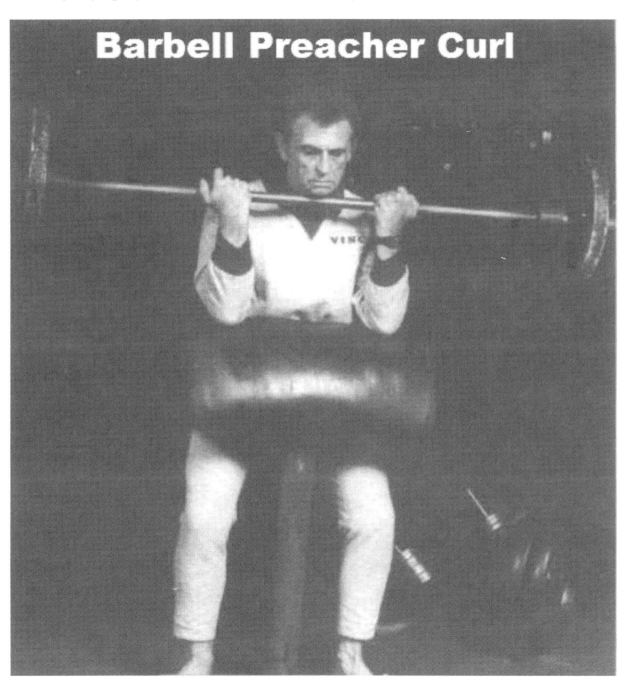

Exercise 2 – Reverse Preacher Curl.

For High Bicep. This exercise is the same as the previous one except your body position is reversed. That is your stomach is against the slanted side of the preacher bench and your upper arms are against the vertical side. Keep your upper arms vertical and curl the bar up under your chin, getting a strong contraction at the top of the movement.

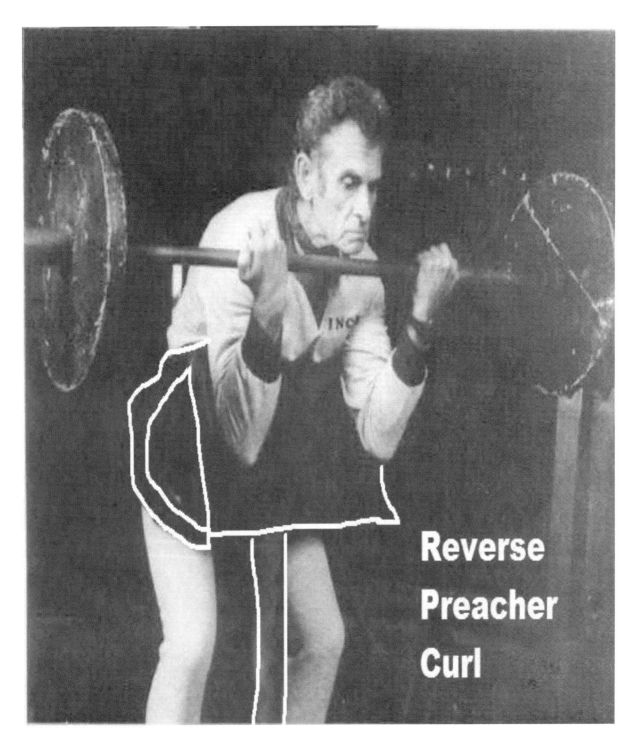

Reverse Preacher Curl

Exercise 3 – Alternate Incline Curls.

For the Middle Bicep. Lay back on the incline bench, keep your chin on your chest, knees slightly bent. Curl your left dumbbell first, keeping your elbow back. As the dumbbell comes up, lean to that side, look at the weight, and forceably contract the bicep when the weight touches the front deltoid. When lowering the left dumbbell, curl the right one, using the same techniques. If you cannot complete 12 twelve reps curling the dumbbells alternately, curl them together.

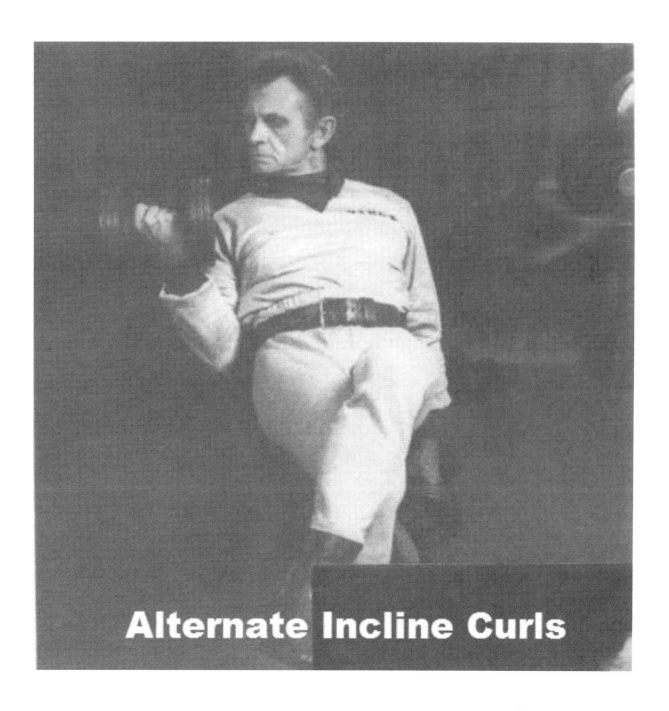

Alternate Incline Curls

Exercise 4 – Seated Dumbbell Curls.

For the Middle and High part of the Biceps. Seated on a flat bench curl your dumbbells together to the shoulders keeping elbows back. The palms face in at the bottom of the curl and up at the top.

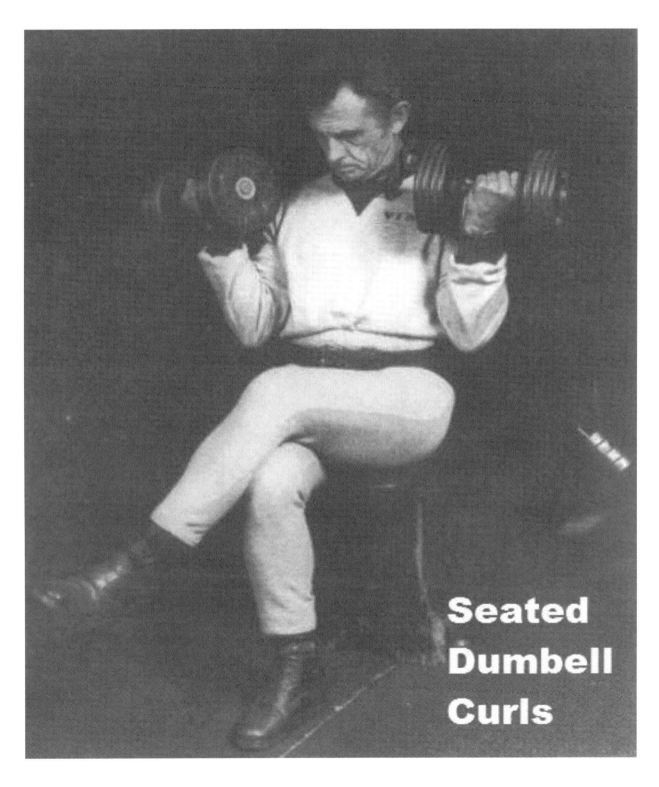

Seated Dumbell Curls

Forearms

Exercise 1 – Barbell Wrist Curl.

For the Belly of Forearm. Place a 10" block under one end of the bench, and sit straddling the bench and facing the low end. Keep your elbows pushed down against the bench, and use your knees to keep them in, so they don't slip off the bench. Allow your barbell to roll down to finger tips, then flex the wrist and keeping the thumb under, grip the bar tightly in the top position. Let the wrist bend backward slowly and open the fingers so that the bar rolls down to finger tips again to start the next rep.

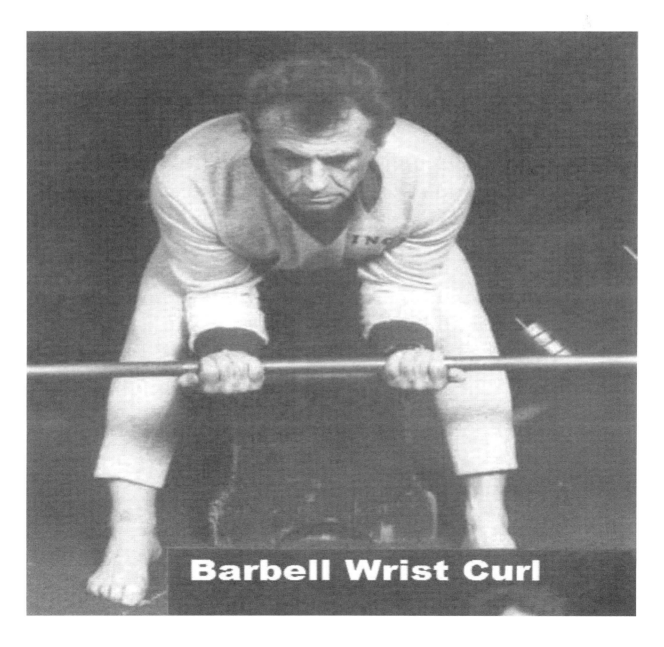

Barbell Wrist Curl

Exercise 2 – Reverse Curl, Body Drag Style.

For the Upper and Outer part of the Forearm. Perform this curl with an overhand grip and thumbs on top of the bar. Curl the bar from the thighs to the upper chest, keeping the elbows back, so that the bar touches the body all the time as it is curled up and lowered down.

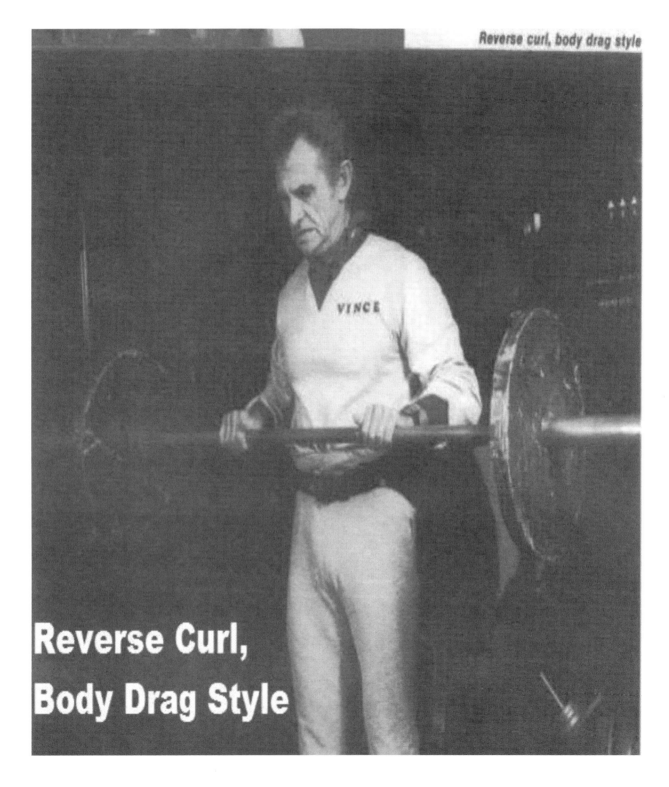

Reverse curl, body drag style

Reverse Curl, Body Drag Style

Exercise 3 – Zottman Curls.

This Exercise Affects 3 Three Different Aspects of the Forearm and Biceps. Hold two dumbbells at your sides. Starting with the left hand, turn the palm out and curl the dumbbell out to the side, up, lean to that side, look at the weight, and forcibly contract the bicep with your right hand, timing your curls so that the left hand is coming down as the right hand goes up. One curl with each arm counts as one rep.

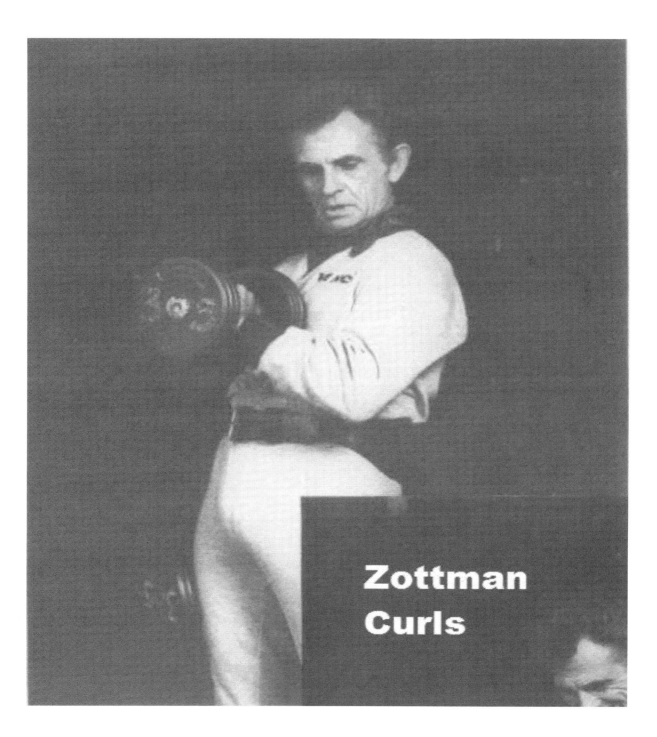

Exercise 4 – Thumbs Up Dumbbell Curl.

For the Upper Outer part of the Forearm. Curl two dumbbells together from the sides of the thighs with the thumbs up, until the ends of the dumbbells touch the front deltoids. Keep the elbows tight to the sides throughout the movement. This completes your routine for Day 2.

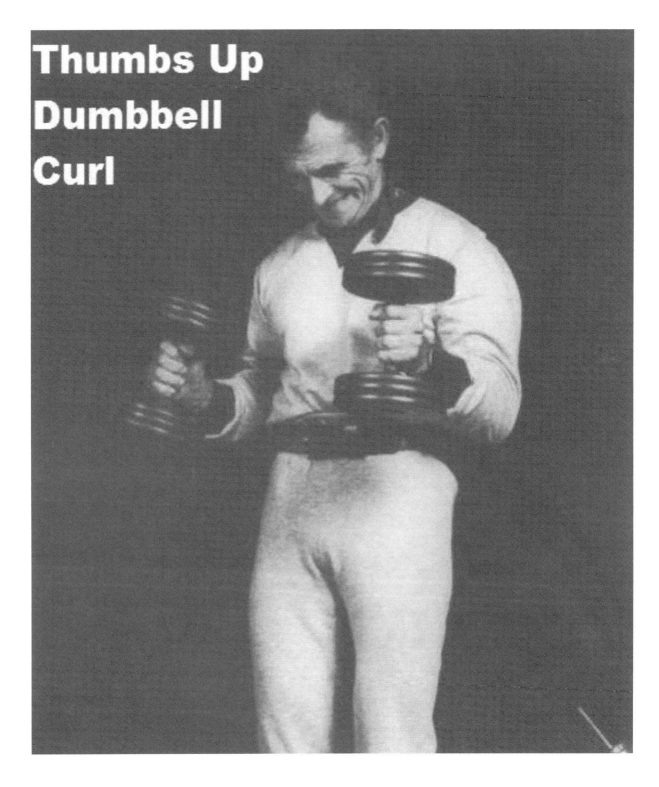

Day 3 – Thighs

Exercise 1 – Sissy Squat.

For the High Thigh Fibres, produces a Longer Look. Hold a barbell in front of your shoulders in the clean position. Place your heels on a 2"× 4" block, 24" apart, and toes wider than the heels. The sissy squat is three separate movements, each performed 4 four repetitions. The first is to bend your knees and lower yourself, but keep your body in a straight line between the knees and shoulders, don't bend at the hip joint. Go down as far as you can and return to the erect position four times. The second part is to sit down on your heels as a starting position, then as you start to rise, drive your hips forward, so that your body is in a straight line from knees to shoulders but the knees are still bent. Do not attempt to come to a full standing position when you reach this stage, sit down on your heels again and repeat four repetitions. The third part is a combination of the first and second part done consecutively. Drop down until you reach the bottom position as you did in part one, then sit on your heels, drive your hips forward until you are in a straight line from knees to shoulders, then stand erect. This is one rep, repeat four times. The sissy squat is the exercise that will give your thighs the champion's look. I regard as being so important that I have written an entire course on it, which you may obtain by writing to me.

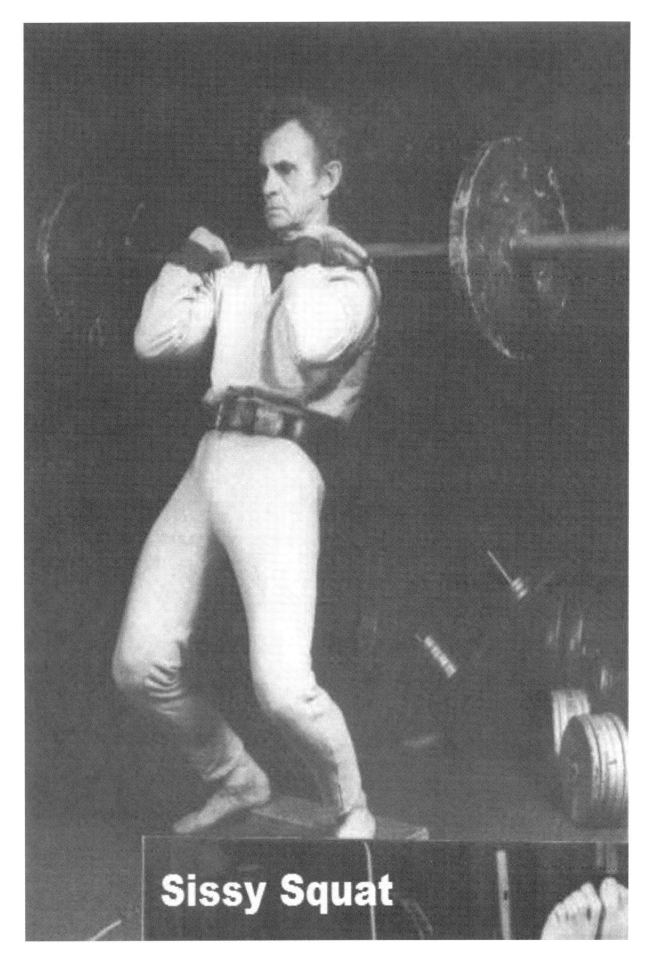

Sissy Squat

Exercise 2 – Power Leg Curl.

For the Hamstrings. Lie on your stomach on the leg curl machine with your heels under the roller, and your toes pointed out. Push up with your arms so that your chest is off the table. Let the body drop, and at the same time curl your heels to the hips, keeping the toes pointed out. Lower the heels slowly back to the starting position.

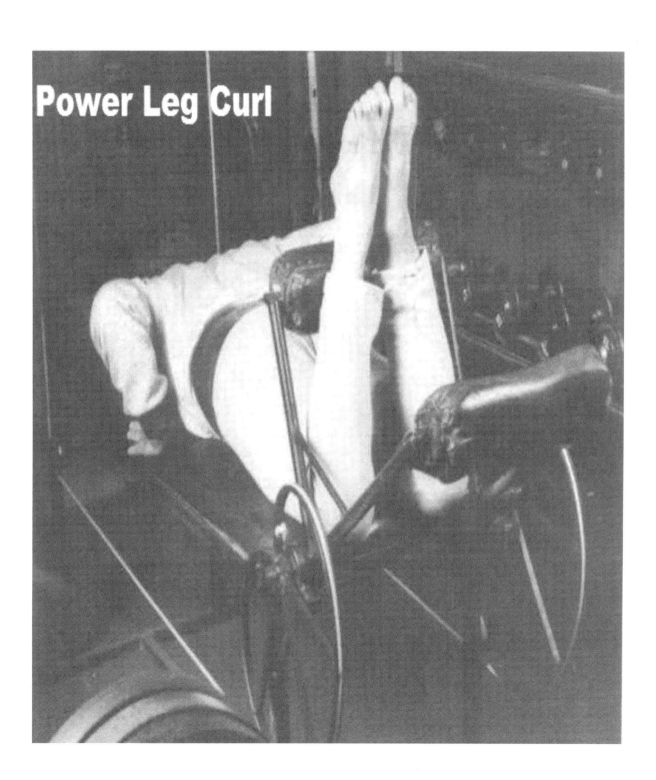

Exercise 3 – Wide Stance Frog Squat.

For the Outer Thigh Curve. Hold the barbell across the front of your shoulders in the clean position. Take a wide plia stance and point your toes outward as far as possible. Keeping your back straight, squat down to a deep position. Do not lean forward when you squat or rise. If your ankles are stiff, you may have to use a block under your heels.

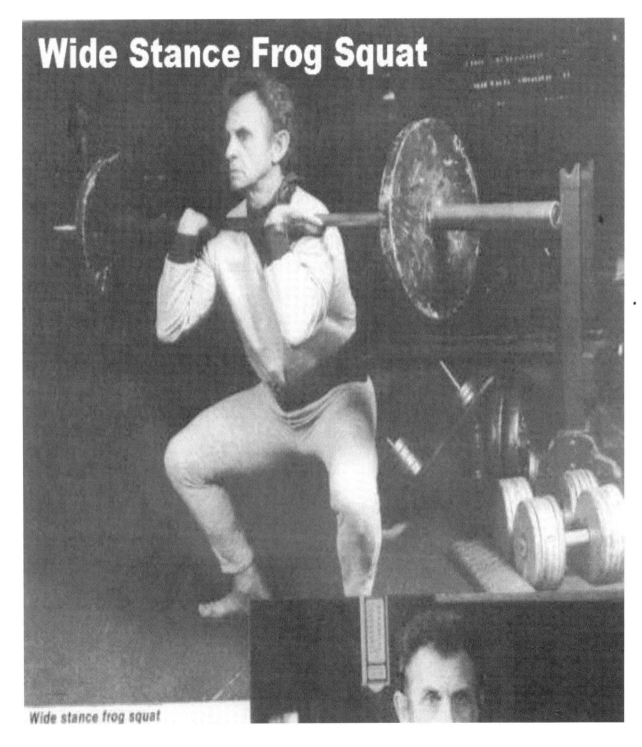

Wide stance frog squat

Exercise 4 – Power Leg Extensions.

For the Front of the Thighs. Sit on the thigh extension table with your hands grasping the sides of the table as far back as you can reach, and the feet hooked under the roller. Straighten your legs, and at the same time lay back to assist. Return slowly to the starting position.

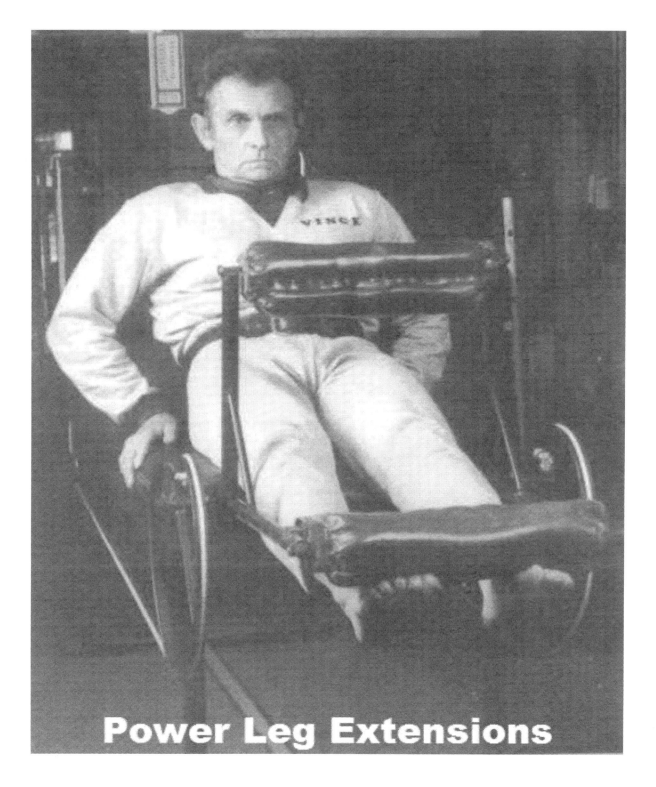

Power Leg Extensions

Calves

Exercise 1 – Seated Heel Raise.

For the Soleus Muscle to give your Calves Width. Perform all your calf exercises with your shoes off. Sit with your feet parallel and 3"apart, knees under the pad, hands grasping the sides of the seat. Lower your heels as far as possible, then, as you raise them lean forward. Get as high on your toes as possible, but above all keep the weight centered on the big toe. Remember to do 20 twenty reps on each calf exercise, instead of the usual twelve.

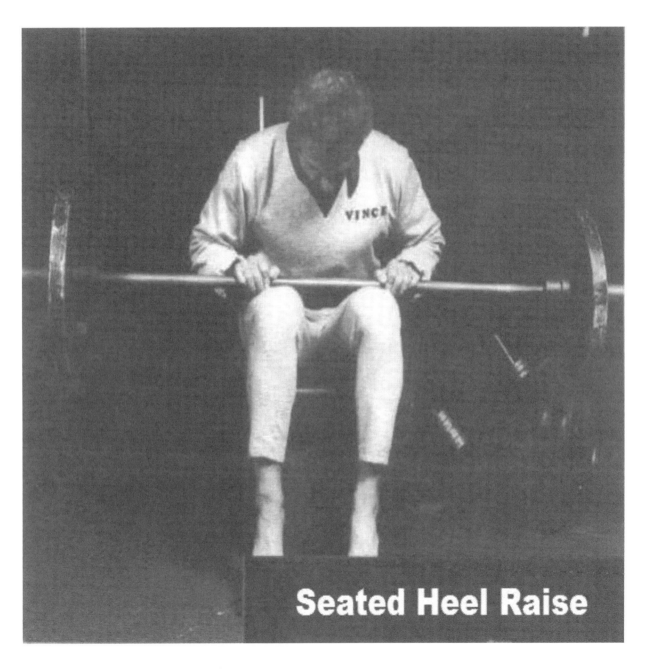

Seated Heel Raise

Exercise 2 – Standing Heel Raise.

For the Inside of the Calf. Get in position on your calf machine, with the feet parallel and the knees locked but slightly bent. Rise up on your toes as high as possible, keeping the weight on the big toe. Lower your heels slowly and try to touch them to the floor. Don't rush through this exercise, use a smooth pumping pace.

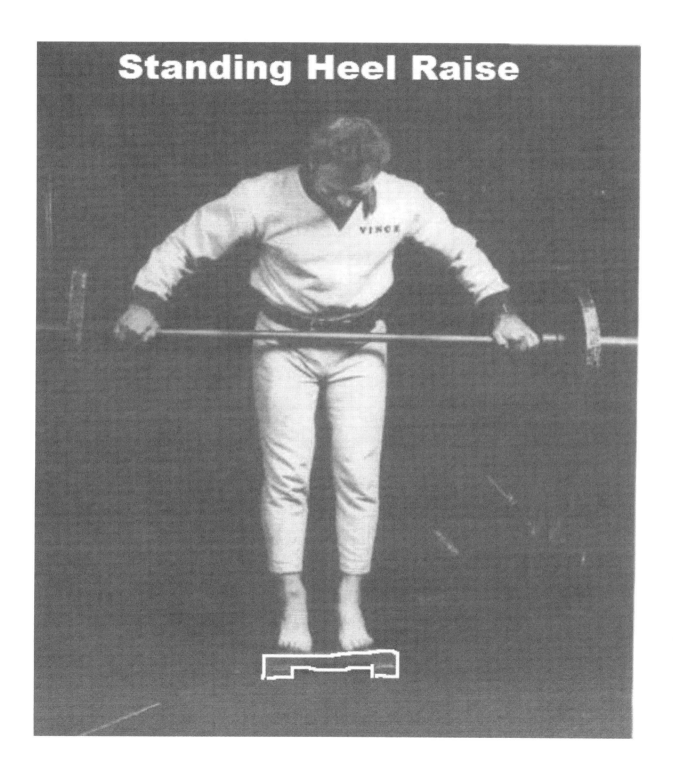

Exercise 3 – Toe Press on the Leg Press Machine.

This is a Stretching Exercise for the High part of the Calf. Lying on your back under the leg press machine, brace your thighs with your hands, and press the weight up with your toes, keeping the pressure on the big toe. Keep your knees locked and your feet parallel, about four inches apart. Lower the weight by letting the ankle bend and the toes point down as far as possible.

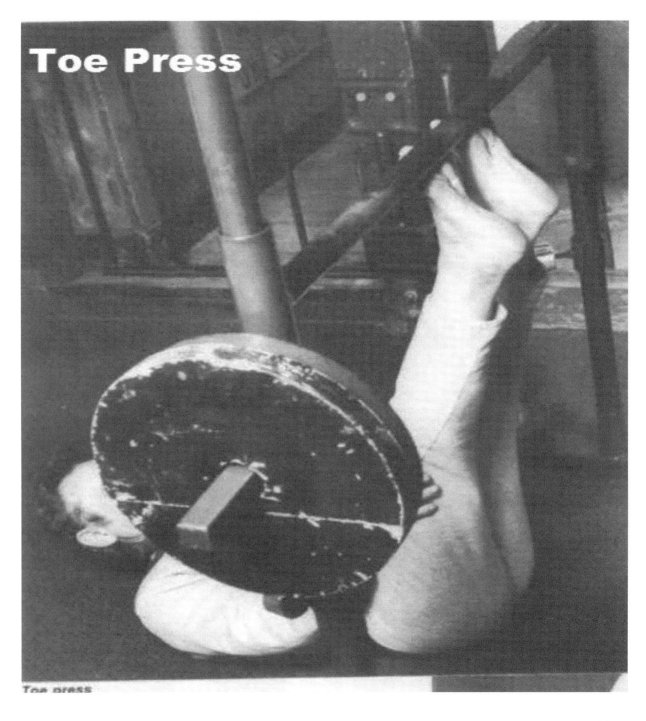

Toe press

Exercise 4 –Hack Slide Heel Raise.

This is a Peak Contraction Exercise to Define the Calf. Face the hack machine with the carriage held against your stomach. Again the feet are parallel about four inches apart. The knees are kept slightly bent throughout the movement. Rise on the toes as high as possible and perform a double contraction at the top of the movement before lowering the heels to the platform. This completes your exercises for Day 3.

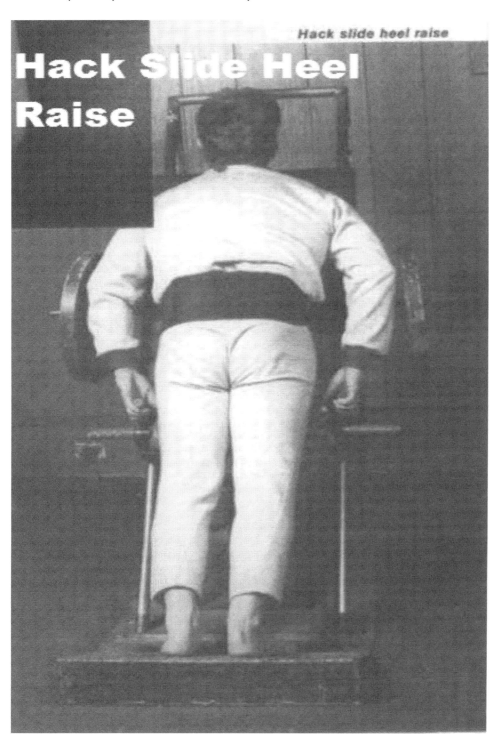

What You Should Eat.

The following is your nutritional program to go with this exercise program. It will provide the materials your body needs to grow at the fastest possible rate. Every three hours, drink six raw eggs, beaten first in a blender, then mixed with half and half separately. Do not mix milk in the blender. With this drink, take 10 Liver tablets, 3 Amino Lysine tablets, 1 Vitamin E, 1 Vitamin B Complex, 1 Chelated Mineral, 1 PABA, and 1 Zinc tablet. The remainder of your diet is Rare Steak and Salad with vinegar and herb dressing. Take 30 Kelp tablets and 1500 milligrams of Vitamin C spread out through the day. The eggs and supplements represent a heavy schedule, and you may have to work into it slowly to have your body accept it. Every three to five days, if you feel weak, eat a total carbohydrate meal to replenish your glycogen reserves.

News from Vince

As I was writing these new courses I was trying to think of what more I could do to help my students achieve the results they want so badly. As most of you know, I have been in this business for nearly 40 years, and have trained literally thousands of stars. Now it is my goal to help as many people as possible. I will make available everything I have learned for the benefit of those who sincerely want results. For this reason I am making the following services available.

1. A complete line of supplements including glandular and synergistic vitamins to give your body the highest level of nutrition. These are NOT products similar to the ones you would find in a health food store. I have used them for years, but have not offered them for sale before.

2. A twelve month course I call the Master Course that gives you twelve different exercise routines and diets that will take you from square one to top shape in one year, without mistakes and setbacks.

3. Finally, I have achieved something I have planned for years. I have made arrangements with a local motel a block away from my gym, so that you can come here and train under my personal supervision for a week or two, or whatever time you wish. You will receive your exercise and nutritional program from me personally.

For information on any of these services or a free catalogue, write to me at:

Vince's Gym

Mail Order Department

11262 Ventura Blvd.

North Hollywood

California, 91604

U.S.A

Please do not phone, I'm just too busy to take phone calls. Thank you for ordering this course, and the very best of health and happiness.

Yours truly

Vince Gironda

Vince Gironda

Made in the USA
Columbia, SC
01 September 2024

41398893R00024